Break Your Sugar Addiction

Why (and how to) Break Free From Your Sugar Habit

RON KNESS

ISBN-13: 978-1541232181

ISBN-10: 1541232186

Contents

Disclaimer

This publication is for informational purposes only and is not intended as medical advice. Medical advice should always be obtained from a qualified medical professional for any health conditions or symptoms associated with them.

Every possible effort has been made in preparing and researching this material. We make no warranties with respect to the accuracy, applicability of its contents or any omissions.

Use caution when beginning a new nutrition, diet, or fitness program. Not all health programs are suitable for everyone.

Check with your doctor before you begin!

Introduction

If you've been struggling with your weight and have what is commonly coined a 'sweet tooth', you are not alone. Many people are drawn to sweet things for a number biological, neurological, and sociological reasons.

Sweetness is one of the first tastes we can register on our

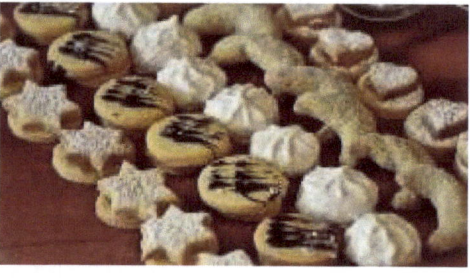

tongue as an infant. The sweetness releases dopamine, a feel good neurotransmitter in the brain. When we are young, our parents try to curb our sweet consumption by giving us sugary foods only as a reward. They become associated with feeling good and being good, so that as we get older, we reward ourselves with sweet treats, often at the expense of our health.

And as the common saying goes, 'forbidden fruits often taste the sweetest'. Sugar, desserts, and items with simple carbohydrates (like soda – one of the worst) can easily start to become a normal part of a teen's or young person's diet once they are allowed to make their own food choices.

Recent studies trying to account for the obesity epidemic that has arisen in the past 40 years, despite the emphasis on a low fat diet, are now turning more and more to looking at sugar and high-carbohydrate foods as the culprit in weight gain, not the consumption of dietary fat. What they have found has shocked them.

A study released in 2007 revealed that for laboratory rats, sugar was more addictive than crack cocaine.

This has led to an all-new body of research on the addictive nature of sugar consumption, with startling results. There is indeed an addictive component to sweet consumption, for a number of reasons. In this guide, we will be outlining sugar addiction, its causes and effects. Then we will be exploring ways to break your sugar addiction to improve your health and live a more balanced lifestyle free from the need for 'sugar fixes'.

Let's get started by discussing the addictive nature of sugar consumption.

Is Sugar More Addictive Than Crack Cocaine?

The original research back in August 2007 that sparked the comparison between sugar being more addictive than crack cocaine was published in the journal **PLOS One**, a publication of the non-profit Public Library of Science.

In the study, 94% of rats who were allowed to choose between sugar water and cocaine chose the sugar. Even rats who were addicted to cocaine quickly switched their preference to sugar once it was offered as a choice. The rats were also more willing to work for sugar than for the cocaine, a 'reward' system which made them crave the sugar even more, leading to addiction, and difficulty when sugar was withdrawn.

Another shocking finding of the study was a cross-tolerance and a cross-dependence between sugars and addictive drugs. For example, lab animals with a long history of sugar consumption actually became tolerant or desensitized to the pain-relieving effects of the potent and addictive painkiller morphine.

The more sugar we get, the more we want, leading to a vicious cycle of craving and satisfaction, back to craving when the 'fix' wears off.

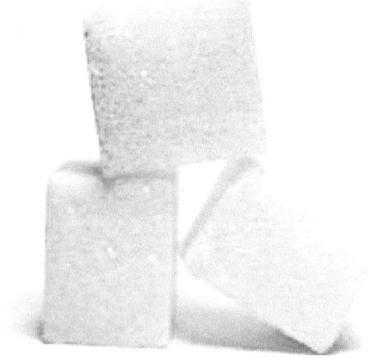

The highs and lows of blood sugar can lead to metabolic syndrome, characterized in part by high blood sugar, high cholesterol and high triglycerides (a form of cholesterol), insulin resistance, pre-diabetes, and Type 2 diabetes. These conditions have now been found in the U.S. in children as young as 18 months, even though they are normally associated with people over 40.

Sugar increases your insulin levels, which can lead to:

- High blood pressure and high cholesterol

- Heart disease

- Diabetes

- Weight gain

- Premature aging

And above all, more cravings for more sugar.

One other thing to note about the study was they tested dopamine levels in relation to the artificial sweetener saccharin (Sweet'n'Low®) as well and got the same result as for sugar. You can read the study abstract here: https://www.ncbi.nlm.nih.gov/pubmed/17668074 and the full study here: http://journals.plos.org/plosone/article?id=10.1371/journal.pone.0000698

After this ground-breaking, study, more researchers sought to study the harmful effects of sugar on the body, and in particular, its addictive nature.

A study published in the *Journal of Neuroscience* in August 2011 showed that dopamine levels paired with other chemical changes in the brain related to the amino acid glutamate (as in monosodium glutamate) affected both levels sugar and cocaine use, but also created a great mental association between reward and the addictive substance. It also demonstrated a clear correlation with increased use of both substances, and with eating disorders. This study could pave the way for more effective interventions for sugar and cocaine addicts and those with a range of eating disorders and obesity issues.

An interesting study published in the journal *Biological Psychiatry* in 2013 titled, "Dual roles of dopamine in food-and-drug seeking: the drive-reward paradox," shows that dopamine produces both a drive for that feel good factor, and a physical need for further reward. Why this should be the case and occurring in the exact same spot in the brain could go a long way towards explaining overeating and other food-related disorders, and drug addiction.

The extreme effects of sugar on the brain might also go a long way toward explaining cognitive impairment, dementia, and Alzheimer's disease, which is more common in women and is linked to sugar consumption.

The study authors conclude there is some in-built link between food and reward, and brain stimulation and reward. They also point to further study of the 'satiety' hormone leptin, which triggers the sensation that a person is full after eating. Studies related to artificial sweeteners show they have a harmful impact on leptin, and insulin, thus leading to food cravings and in the case of leptin, to abdominal obesity.

Another key study points to the role of stress in our eating habits. In the journal *Minerva endocrinologica*, a study published in September 2013 titled, "Stress and eating behaviors," has shown that not all obesity is the same, but rather, can be stress-driven, with stress affecting food choices, in particular, high sugar ones, which may possess addictive qualities.

Stress is an important factor in the development of addiction and in relapse when a person is trying to recover from it. Stress may also contribute to an increased risk for obesity and other metabolic diseases. Uncontrollable stress changes eating patterns, and the tendency to consume more sweets. Over time, this could lead to changes in the brain and behavior, resulting in increasingly compulsive behavior, in which the person 'just can't seem to help themselves'.

The chemical changes seem to center on the hypothalamus, pituitary and adrenal glands, and affect glucose metabolism (blood sugar), insulin sensitivity, and other appetite-related hormones and chemicals. These changes can even alter the wiring in the brain, with dopamine becoming connected to the stress and motivation circuits in the brain. This can result in an increase in cravings for sweets, a greater reward mentality, and an increase in weight, which leads to more cravings, stress and need for reward. The study shows that those with a sugar addiction are 5 times more likely to 'binge eat' than those who don't.

Now that we understand why researchers have labelled sugar as more addictive than crack cocaine in reference to laboratory animals, let's look at other reasons why sugar can be so addictive to humans.

Why Is Sugar So Addictive In People?

There are a number of reasons why sugar can be so addictive to humans. The first is that sugar is tasty and can make even sour foods more palatable. We discover sweetness as infants when we are fed applesauce and other fruits or given juice.

Unless the juice is 100% natural, it will often contain high fructose corn syrup (HFCS), which as the name suggests, is high in sugar (fructose, that is, fruit sugar). HFCS can trigger bloating, belly fat and weight gain. It can also trigger cravings for even more sweet things.

Researchers speculate that the sweet receptors, that is, two protein receptors located on the tongue, which evolved in early humans, have not adapted to the high sugar lifestyle of the modern world. The 'eat like a caveman' focus of the Paleo diet, which is low in carbohydrates, might be onto something.

Eating anything sweet will release the feel-good neurotransmitter dopamine, forging a link between eating sugary foods and enhanced mood and well-being, however temporary before the sugar high becomes a sugar low. The lows can leave you feeling depressed, listless and 'down', so a person will give themselves a 'pick-me-up', usually in the form of a sweet treat.

Modern diets are much higher in sugar, HFCS, and foods that might seem to be healthy forms of sugar, such as honey, than our ancestors.

The abnormally high stimulation of our tongue receptors due to our sugar-rich diets generates excessive reward signals in the brain. These excessive signals have the potential to override normal self-control mechanisms, and thus lead overeating of sugar and from there to addiction.

Low fat, but high sugar

The low fat diet craze and introduction of artificial sweeteners for commercial use in the last few decades have resulted in unprecedented levels of obesity in the U.S. and many countries in the world that adopt a Westernized diet high in what can be termed junk (processed fast) food.

If you remove the fat from food, you need to replace it with something that will maintain its flavor. Added sugar, artificial sweeteners and 'flavorings' have been added due to the focus on a low fat diet. One of the few people who bucked this trend, as far back as the early 1970s, was Dr. Atkins.

Atkins argued that the best way to lose weight was to eat diets low in processed carbohydrates, like bread, cake, cookies and so on, and eat a diet rich in protein, leafy vegetables and healthy fats such as those found in nuts and lean meats. For decades, he was laughed at, until a growing body of weight loss success stories supported his claims.

Another doctor who was laughed out of his profession was John Yudkin, who in the UK in 1972, published his book ***Pure, White and Deadly***, about the dangerous effects of sugar.

In the book he pointed out that until the emergence of what could be termed the convenience food industry in the 1850s and the wider availability of sugar, there were far fewer health issues such as high cholesterol (in particular high triglycerides) and Type 2 diabetes.

Ludkin was founder of the nutrition department at the University of London's Queen Elizabeth College, so he was clearly an expert in his field. However, he was no match for the food industry in general and the sugar industry in particular. His theories were accurate, but observational, and therefore not presented with the degree of rigorous clinical data that might have silenced his critics.

Ludkin was not only ostracized from medical conferences, his publications were omitted from the collections of the few he did attend and he was publicly attacked to the point where many other researchers dared not voice any criticism of sugar for fear of getting the same treatment.

The reason for the attacks? The food industry was on the low-fat train and could only sell more if they used more sugar to replace the fat.

Now proponents of the anti-sugar movement, such as **Robert Lustig** in the U.S., can see that Ludkin was right in many respects. Sugar has a huge impact on certain hormones that weren't even discovered at the time that Ludkin was working, but that he could see from his observational studies were significantly impacted by sugar consumption, leading to obesity, heart disease and more.

The reward mentality

Another key reason for sugar addition, or carbohydrate addiction, as the Hellers, also proponents of the low-carb lifestyle, have termed it, is the reward mentality. Parents would bribe us with dessert if we ate all our food. We would get a sweet treat if we were 'good'. No birthday seems complete without a cake, or cupcakes, to the point where many schools in the U.S. started to ban them, and birthday celebrations in general, over alarm at the growing rate of obesity amongst young people, currently around 33%.

The end of year holidays, such as Halloween, Thanksgiving and

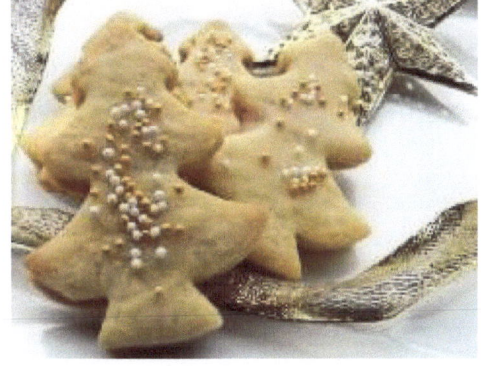

Christmas, feature sweet foods and dessert heavily, from candy and desserts to sweet potato casserole, stuffing, pumpkin pie, cranberry sauce and other high-carb foods. Americans take the best of nature's bounty and douse it in HFCS, white sugar or brown sugar. Holidays are supposed to be a happy time, so these special foods are equated with feeling good and rewards.

That reward mentality spills over into daily life. If we work hard, we often reward ourselves with food, such as a snack, a takeaway meal on the way home, ordering in, or dining out. Many of these foods have hidden sugar and/or artificial sweeteners.

This can lead to a cycle of addiction, in more ways than one. Ever wonder why you are hungry again only a couple of short hours after you've stuffed yourself with a good meal? It's probably the carbs. As the Hellers explain in their carbohydrate addicts books, the level of insulin we release after eating is in direct relation to the amount of carbs in the meal we have consumed. In most cases, it should be in balance.

For simple carbs like sugar addicts, however, it is not just in relation to what you have just eaten, but possibly as many as your 4 previous meals, so that the more sugar you eat, the more insulin you produce. If you keep on pumping out a lot of insulin, sooner or later you will develop insulin-related disorders, such as insulin resistance, and eventually, Type 2 diabetes. This form of diabetes is increasingly common among children, compared with the autoimmune Type 1 diabetes, and thus seems to indicate that there is something seriously out of balance with our diets and it needs to be addressed. That imbalance is most likely the high amount of sugar, artificial sweeteners, and sugar substitutes being put into everything from cereal to salad dressing.

These days, it is easy to be fooled by the foods you eat in relation to the amount of sugar you are consuming. Let's look at the reasons for this in the next chapter.

Don't Be Fooled By Natural-Sounding Sugar Substitutes

A recent trend in the food industry has been 'natural' sugar substitutes that are supposed to be healthier for you than sugar. In many cases, these are just as bad for you as processed white table sugar. In some instances, they can even be worse.

Sugar is derived from 2 sources:

- Sugar Cane

- Sugar Beet

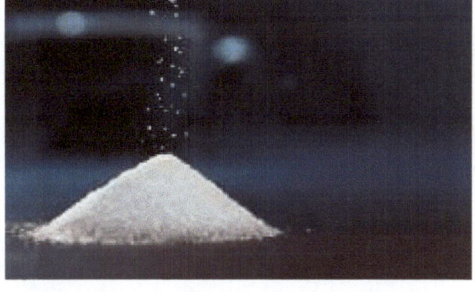

The detailed story of sugar at the **National Geographic website** (http://ngm.nationalgeographic.com/2013/08/sugar/cohen-text) makes for hair-raising reading if you are at all concerned about human right and/or your health. They argue that the entire age of exploration was at least in part triggered by European desire to grow more sugar. The slave trade was at least in part founded by the sugar cane industry.

Studies show that sugar consumption increased exponentially from around 7 pounds a year per person before the sugar race to more than 100 pounds after it in the UK alone. This alarming trend actually caused some people to call for it to be banned, or subject to the same regulation and harsh taxation as alcohol and tobacco, which the English government also tried to have banned when it started being imported from the American colonies.

Barbados was one of the first 'sugar islands' and cultivation and production in the Caribbean became so great that almost the whole of many islands was given over to it. The surplus grew so great, the rum trade was founded.

Fast forward to the modern world, and people have become more aware of how bad white sugar can be for them in terms of their teeth, weight and health, leading to an all-new emphasis on healthier sweeteners such as artificial substitutes and natural substitutes for it.

A growing body of research has shown that artificial sweeteners like Splenda®, NutraSweet® and saccharin are NOT harmless and can cause severe side effects, including diabetes, brain issues and even death.

Natural sweeteners may sound attractive, but they can be just as dangerous as sugar, if not more so. In terms of the body's metabolism, it does not see any difference and processes it just as it would sugar. Honey is therefore just as bad, brown sugar and molasses even more so. The sugar turns to 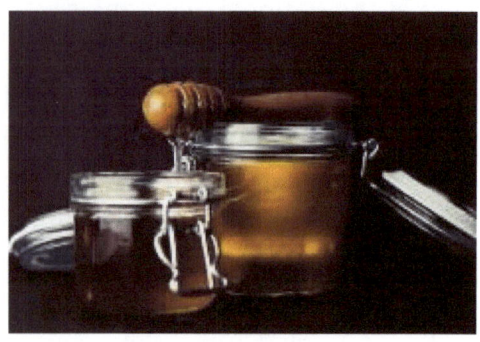 alcohol in the blood in some cases, leading to liver damage.

The biggest issue is that of food labeling. Even smart shoppers reading labels and trying to make smart choices for their families can be fooled.

Look at all of the names for what is essentially sugar in the pre-packaged foods sitting on store shelves:

- Barley Malt Extract Syrup
- Brown Rice Syrup
- Brown Sugar
- Corn Sugar
- Corn Sweetener
- Corn Syrup, or Corn Syrup Solids
- Crystalline Fructose
- Dehydrated Cane Juice
- Dextrin
- Dextrose
- Evaporated Cane Juice
- Fructose
- Fruit Juice Concentrate
- Glucose
- High-Fructose Corn
- Honey
- Invert Sugar (golden syrup)
- Lactose
- Maltodextrin
- Malt syrup
- Maltose
- Maple Syrup
- Molasses
- Raw Sugar
- Rice Syrup
- Sucrose Sorghum Syrup
- Syrup (golden syrup, dark syrup, light syrup)
- Treacle
- Turbinado Sugar

Let's just look at few of the ones at the top of this list:

Barley Malt Extract - full of gluten and basically the same as eating Metamucil fiber. Side effects include:

- Nausea
- Heart Burn
- Mild Abdominal Cramps
- Severe Abdominal Pain
- Bloating
- Vomiting
- Diarrhea
- Dehydration
- Gas/Flatulence
- Intestinal Blockage

It's only advantage is that in lab mice, it has less impact on blood sugar than table sugar.

Brown Rice Syrup - also called Rice Malt Syrup

According to the Sydney University Glycemic Index (GI) database, brown rice syrup has a glycemic index of 98, which is extremely high. It is much higher than table sugar (GI of 60-70) and higher than almost any other sweetener on the market. If you eat rice syrup, then it is highly likely to lead to rapid spikes in blood sugar, making it dangerous for those with diabetes. In addition, a lot of it is contaminated with the heavy metal arsenic.

Acute or immediate symptoms of a toxic level of exposure to arsenic may include the following:

- Vomiting
- Diarrhea
- Abdominal pain
- Dark urine

- Dehydration
- Heart problems
- Hemolysis (destruction of red blood cells)
- Dizziness
- Delirium
- Shock
- Death

Arsenic can damage every major organ of the body even in small doses. Brown rice syrup is found in crackers and cookies. High levels of arsenic have also been found in protein drinks such as Muscle Milk, leading to a much greater risk of poisoning.

Fructose, and High Fructose Corn Syrup (HFCS)

Fructose means fruit sugar. HFCS has got a higher amount of fructose, making it sweeter and therefore even more dangerous because of its addictive nature as well as its alarming side effects.

HFCS has been linked to:

- Metabolic syndrome
- Insulin resistance
- Diabetes
- Poor blood glucose control
- Damage to the immune system
- Accelerated aging
- Mercury poisoning
- Obesity
- Heart health issues

The average American consumes around 300 grams of carbohydrates per day, around 22 teaspoons of sugar, which adds up to around 175 pounds of sugar per year. The American Heart Association recommends that most women get no more than 100 calories a day of added sugar from any source, and that most men get no more than 150 calories a day of added sugar. That's about 6 teaspoons of added sugar for women and 9 teaspoons for men per day maximum.

For those who say, "But I never touch the sugar bowl!" the truth is that if you don't make your food yourself from scratch, you have no control over the amount of **added** sugar, sweeteners and artificial sweeteners you are consuming.

So what's a person to do if they want to break their sugar addition and wean themselves off what has been termed 'white death'? Let's look at some of the best ways to eliminate sugar from your diet in the next chapter.

How to Reverse Your Sugar Addiction in 15 Days

There are all sorts of sugar detox diets online, but most of them lack any science behind them. In addition, they will not usually support your most likely secondary goal when weaning yourself off sugar, trying to lose weight and keeping it off.

One of the easiest ways to do a sugar detox is to follow a low carb diet such as Atkins. The starting phase of Atkins, the Induction phase, is probably the toughest diet you will ever be on IF you stick to it 100% for the first 2 weeks, BUT the results will be well worth it.

A second way to rid yourself of unwanted sugar, sugar substitutes and artificial sweeteners, all of which the body processes as sugar, is to 'eat clean', that is, cook your food yourself using fresh ingredients in as natural a form as possible. Clean eating means freeing yourself as far as possible from any chemicals in your diet that could be affecting your health adversely. It will usually mean choosing organic if you

can afford to. Otherwise, go to your nearest farmer's market and buy meat and produce from your local producers, since they will be far less likely to be bathed in 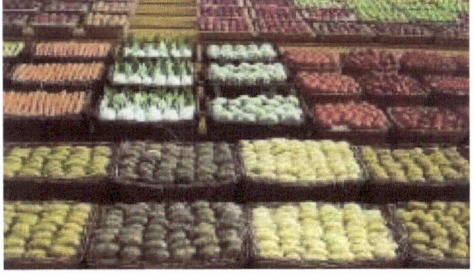 pesticides or full of hormones or genetically modified compared to what you will find in the supermarket.

A clean-eating Atkins diet will help you lose weight and look and feel great, but above all, it will wean you off sugar to the point where you won't crave it any longer. And all in a little over 2 weeks! So let's get started with a simple 15-day sugar detox plan.

DAY 1

Education and Preparation

Today you are going to take your first step of your sugar detox diet by educating yourself about how much sugar is really in the foods you eat, and how to get started making healthier choices.

Learn the Atkins basics

We are suggesting Atkins because it is the most tried and tested low carb diet with the largest number of free resources available, and the recipes are pretty tasty compared with South Beach or Paleo.

Induction allows you only 20 grams of carbs per day, and NO fruit, sugars or sweet treats for these 14 days. How much are 20 grams of carbs? Use the free carb counter available to help you out.

https://files.atkins.com/1501_CarbCounter_Online.pdf

Note: avoid the pre-prepared Atkins foods when looking over the carb counter. Remember that you are eating clean as well as carb counting.

Raid the pantry

Go to your pantry and check the labels in relation to the amount of carbs and the ingredients in each food. Get a red pen if you like to circle those items on the label, and anything else you may not have any idea of what it is. Separate all the food out into too high in carbs or unnatural, that you need to get rid of, and food you can keep.

This may be upsetting if you have just done a big shopping trip, but it is important for several reasons.

- Learn more about the food you have been eating. You didn't become addicted to sugar overnight and once you do your detox, you never want to go back.

- If you have it in the house, you will be tempted to eat it. Out of sight, out of mind.

- If you are an emotional eater, such as when you are under stress, or a binge eater, when you get a sugar craving, you will be at much greater risk of falling off the wagon with your sugar detox program if you don't get them out of the house.

Bundle up all the unopened food and donate to a local food pantry. Get a receipt for your donation if you can, for tax purposes. For opened food, bring it to work or a local community gathering such as a church picnic.

Start menu planning

Look up recipes for Atkins Phase 1. The Atkins 20 "Foodie" Menu plan at https://files.atkins.com/Atkins-20-Foodie-Meal-Plan-5.27.16.pdf is a good starting point provided you ignore the instructions to buy their prepared food and snack bars and eat all natural snacks like celery and carrot sticks. Print out a copy so you can jot down notes as needed. You will be using the Foodie menu because you are also clean eating and will be cooking for yourself on the diet.

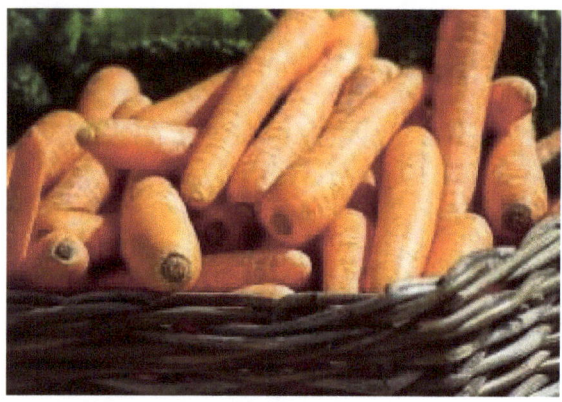

Look at the shopping lists for week 1 and 2 on the last pages of the PDF. If you are going to use any of the suggested salad dressings and sauces, make your own from scratch using low carb recipes for ketchup and barbecue sauce and so on.

If you absolutely can't live without some form of sweetener, use stevia. The **NOW brand** of pure stevia extract is the only one that doesn't have any additional ingredients. Here is a link: http://amzn.to/2hOmPYw. Be careful when first using, since stevia is about 100 times sweeter than sugar, so a tiny bit will go a long way in your sauces.

Edit the shopping list for Week 1 according to your personal tastes. If you don't eat red meat or fish, for instance, swap with lean poultry or tofu.

Note that not ALL foods are created equal.

Some can actually curb your sugar cravings. Add the following foods to your diet each day:

- Avocado

- Broccoli

- Kale

- Spinach

They help regulate blood sugar.

For beverage, drink green tea. For dessert, have a nibble of dark chocolate, such as Lindt 85% or higher. Another good choice would be natural peanut butter on a celery stick, or plain or vanilla 0% Greek-style yogurt.

Go shopping and stick to your list.

Ignore anything that is not on your list for week 1.

Buy chromium picolinate

This supplement has been linked to better blood sugar regulation and can support you during the early days when you are weaning yourself off sugar. Optimal doses appear to be from 200 to 600 micrograms per day. They are usually sold in 200 microgram tablets, such as from **Now Foods** (http://amzn.to/2hNvIPJ). Take it before you eat.

Its effects can last as many as 4 hours even when in contact with stomach acid.

Buy a reliable food scale

If you don't already have one, get an inexpensive **food scale** (http://amzn.to/2i956ax) to help measure your portions.

Start a food diary

Get a small notebook you can carry with you to track your eating and your feelings as you undergo your sugar detox journey.

If you are interested in losing weight through your sugar detox and own a scale, weigh yourself and note that number down in your food diary.

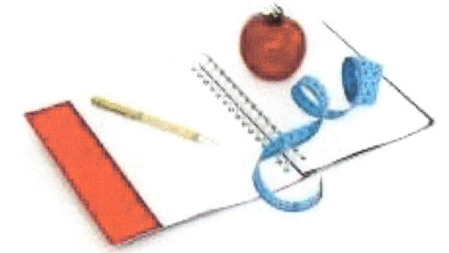

Hopefully you will feel excited to start your new healthy eating plan tomorrow morning.

DAY 2

Today is your big day. Hopefully you will feel excited about starting your new sugar detox program. You might also be in for a big shock. We are betting that many of your favorite 'go to' foods are off the menu, especially in relation to breakfast.

Breakfast for most people tends to be high in carbs, such as cereal, toast and so on. Atkins Induction will be eggs 4 times a week, and breakfast meat or fish for the other 3. Cook your breakfast for the day.

While your breakfast is cooking, organize your snacks and lunch for the day if you work outside the home. Celery and peanut butter will transport well.

Lunch is supposed to be salmon, but if you prefer, you can swap the dinner meal of chicken and eat the salmon hot. Both of the meats can be eaten hot or cold. Don't forget to take your chromium before each meal.

The snack suggests an Atkins ready-made shake, but you can create your own smoothie with unsweetened soy milk or skim milk, peanut butter if you are not allergic, and some dark chocolate shavings.

Eat your:

- Avocado

- Broccoli

- Kale

- Spinach

.. as snacks too. The latter 3 can be raw or cooked.

Journal in your food diary at the end of the day. What did you enjoy? What did you find tough?

Review your menu plans for tomorrow. Plan your substitutions as needed, such as chicken or tofu instead of the steak at dinner, perhaps made into a stir fry.

DAY 3

You should be looking forward to another day working towards your best and healthiest self, free from sugar addition.

Review today's menus as you prepare breakfast and pack up your lunch and snacks. If you are craving sweets, try some green tea with a twist of lemon or lime, or a flavored seltzer.

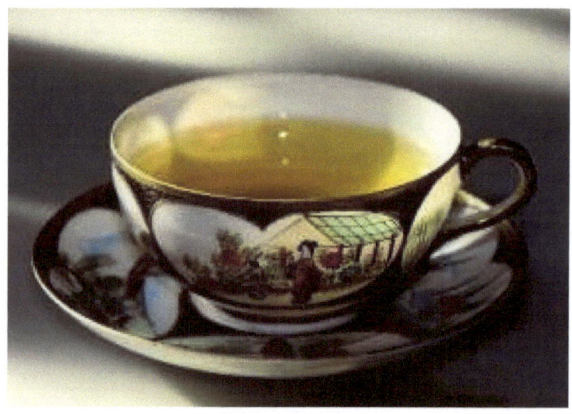

Eat your blood-sugar-regulating vegetables and remember to take your chromium with each meal.

You might be feeling a bit low-energy due to the chemical changes in your body. Try to add some exercise to your day, such as walking around the block after dinner. Exercise boosts energy and enhances mood by increasing dopamine levels naturally without being related to food.

Journal about your day in your food diary.

DAY 4

Today we have some new dishes to look forward to for Day 3 on the menu plan PDF.

Dinner looks a bit sparse, so eat your broccoli, spinach and kale then.

Kale also makes a great snack. Try this recipe, a delicious crispy treat similar to seaweed:

- 10 ounces of fresh kale, washed well

- ½ tsp Kosher salt or other coarse salt

- Non-Stick cooking spray

Preheat your oven to 350ºF.

Remove thick stems from kale and tear the leaves into large pieces. Arrange the leaves in a single layer on a baking sheet.

Spray the kale lightly with non-stick cooking spray and sprinkle with the Kosher salt. Bake in the oven for about 15 minutes until the kale is crisp. Cool the pieces and enjoy them as a healthy snack any time.

Assess the role of stress in your life. You might have had a good couple of days so far. However, if stress has put you under pressure and tempted you to eat forbidden foods, it's time to start looking at natural stress relief methods. Let's start by assessing what stresses you.

List them in your journal, such as your boss, your weight, a difficult relationship and so on.

Write down how you usually cope with that problem. Then try to think of 3 healthy things you could do to solve the issue.

Example: My boss stresses me.

- Take breaks more often.

- Go for a walk at lunch so I don't make bad food choices.

- Use a stop watch to track where my time is going at work so I can be more productive and less stressed.

DAY 5

Examine your protein intake. One of the reasons why a lot of people have dismissed the low carb lifestyle is because it contains a lot of protein, which some say can be very dangerous over time. However, protein is one of the keys to feeling satisfied and not overeating. It's also important for regulating blood sugar and insulin, and curbing cravings.

If you are struggling to make breakfast every morning, start the day with a smoothie made with soy milk and decaf coffee powder, or decaf green tea with yogurt.

Also mix and match meats as needed. If you don't like bacon, eat ham. Aim for low sodium varieties and watch out for salt generally in your diet. It can also cause cravings.

Skip the snack bar listed on the menu and use your broccoli, kale and spinach instead. Enjoy with some homemade ranch dressing or a peanut butter based dressing.

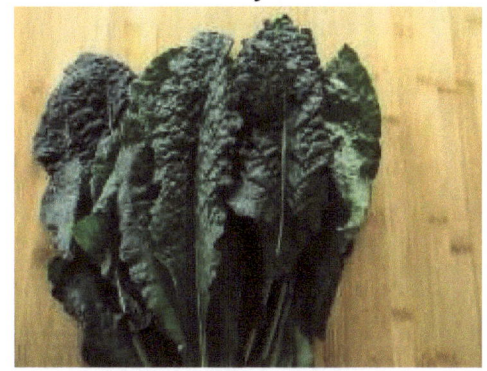

Journal about your eating habits.

DAY 6

Focus on your sleep habits

If you're like most people, once the weekend rolls around, you go into hibernation mode, trying to catch up on lost sleep you might have missed out on during the week, or getting more as you relax and unwind.

The ideal is 8 hours per night, but most busy people get only 6 to 7. Studies have shown that a lack of sleep leaves people open to sugar and carb cravings because they affect your appetite hormones. In human studies, depriving college students of just two hours of the recommended eight hours of sleep led to a rise in hunger hormones, a decrease in appetite-suppressing hormones and strong cravings for sugar and refined carbs.

It also stands to reason that if you are awake, you will be tempted to eat, versus when you are asleep. Eight hours is ideal; try not to get more than 9 hours a night. Try to stick to the same routine even on weekends so you don't get your body clock confused.

If you don't have a regular bedtime, set one and try to stick to it. Note what you have learned in your journal. Set your alarm and get ready for the next day.

DAY 7

Check your menu

Today calls for Atkins frozen chili, but since you are clean eating, you need to cook it yourself from scratch. Try this low carb recipe from the Atkins website. https://www.atkins.com/recipes/super-chili-bowl/620 Make sure you have all of the ingredients in the house. Note that most beans are too high in carbs to be permitted in the Induction phase. Enjoy your daily avocado on the side for a Mexican-style meal.

Go for a walk. It will get you out of the house and boost your energy levels.

Journal in your food diary.

DAY 8

Welcome to the second week of your sugar detox. We are getting to day 7 of the meals from week one and it is time to weigh yourself to see how you are doing with your weight loss goal.

Note that most of the first 5 pounds or so that you lose will be water weight, but if you keep it up, you will start to shed fat too. Weigh yourself and compare numbers.

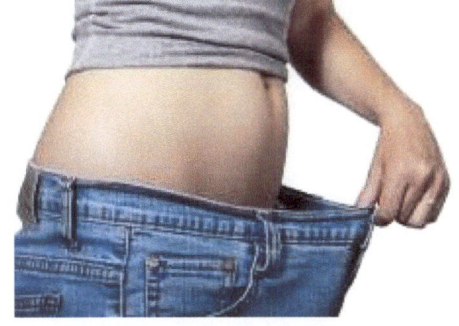

Go shopping for week 2. Again, substitute to suit your tastes and plan to make any sauces and dressings from scratch as far as you can.

Try yoga in order to build strength. A beginner video can show you a range of easy poses (http://eternalspiralbooks.com/40-hatha-yoga-poses-for-beginners) to try.

Journal about your progress and how you feel now that you are breaking the sugar habit and eating clean.

DAY 9

Welcome to Week 2, Day 1 of your Atkins Foodie Meal plan. You can look forward to different dishes and even more weight loss if that is your goal.

Eat your meals for the day, and don't forget to have your chromium before. Use your broccoli, kale and spinach as snacks.

Go for a walk, adding more distance to burn more calories and keep you away from the temptations of food.

Journal about how you feel things are going, and anything you might be struggling with. If there are any issues, what action steps can you take to solve them?

DAY 10

Today is Week 2, Day 2 on the eating plan. Skip the snack bar and eat your additional vegetables.

Today, we are going to look at stress in a bit more detail. Chances are you might be feeling under pressure due to the extreme difference in your eating habits if you were used to turning to sugary foods as a coping mechanism when times became tough.

There are a number of things you can do to relieve stress naturally:

- Exercise

- Learn how to say no

- Make better choices

- Don't try to multitask. Focus on one thing and get it done.

- Spend time with a loved one or friend

Journal about how things are going.

DAY 11

The Week 2, Day 3 menu is tasty and filling. Adjust as needed depending on whether you want hot or cold food and what is easy to take with you to eat outside of your home.

 Learn more about meditation. There are many free resources online. Practice long, deep breathing, focusing on the in and out of your breath for about 5 minutes. http://www.how-to-meditate.org/breathing-meditations

Learn how to meditate and do it for a few minutes each morning and evening. This can help curb cravings and cut the link between mood and food.

Journal about your day.

DAY 12

The Week 2, Day 4 menu doesn't really need any alterations, but use only unsweetened coconut milk and skip the protein powder due to the chemicals. Use yogurt instead.

Learn more about clean eating. Study the Dirty Dozen and Clean 15 information here:
https://www.ewg.org/foodnews/summary.php

The first list is of foods most affected by pesticides, the second those least affected. Print it out or make notes in your journal.

Take a walk after dinner. Add more steps to burn more calories and boost mood.

DAY 13

The Week 2, Day 5 menu

Today's dinner menu calls for frozen shrimp scampi. Make a stir fry instead, or shrimp cocktail if you wish, or substitute any other protein you enjoy.

Check your sleep levels again. Are you getting a full 8 hours?

Study stress management online. There are many free resources that can help, such as the one at: https://thiswayup.org.au/how-we-can-help/courses/coping-with-stress/

Try yoga in order to build strength. A beginner's video can show you a range of easy poses (http://eternalspiralbooks.com/40-hatha-yoga-poses-for-beginners/) to try.

Journal as needed about how well things are going and how you feel.

DAY 14

Review the Week 2, Day 6 menu.

There are no clean eating substitutions needed. Enjoy your extra vegetables any time.

Go for a walk today. Practice a stress management technique you enjoy, such as reading a book for 5 minutes.

Journal about your experiences.

DAY 15

Congratulations! You've made it. If you've stuck to Atkins 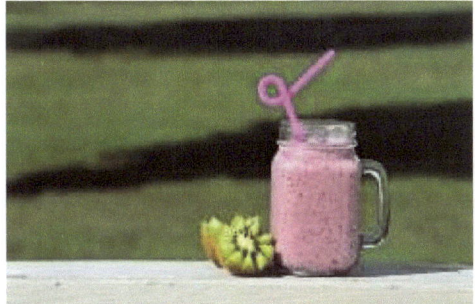 Induction and been eating clean, you've gone 14 days without sugar. You've also gone 2 weeks without a lot of chemicals in your food. Enjoy your meals today. Swap the ready-made shake on the menu for a homemade smoothie.

How do you feel? Journal about it.

How much do you weigh? Did you lose any weight?

Now you have a choice. Do you want to stick to Induction for another couple of weeks, or go to Phase 2?

Phase 2 will allow up to 40 grams of carbs a day. You can find the menu plan here: https://files.atkins.com/Atkins-40-Foodie-Meal-Plan.pdf

Adjust as needed with your own tastes and the clean eating rules in mind.

Not sure which to choose? Decide based on how much weight you want to lose. If it is more than 40 pounds, stay on Induction. If you've really struggled, also stay on Induction to reduce your risk of falling back into old habits.

Educate yourself about healthy fats. A good article on fats is at: https://www.atkins.com/how-it-works/library/articles/good-fats. Aim for olive oil, canola and peanut. Fat is not a bad word with Atkins because it makes you full, balances your blood sugar and is necessary for cell health. Along with protein, eat good fats at every meal, including avocados, nuts and seeds.

Now that you've gotten though your 14- day sugar detox and clean eating routine, we hope you are feeling and looking great. If you want to return to relatively normal eating habits once more, however, there are several important things you need to know about carbohydrates. Let's look at them in the next chapter.

Important Issues With Carbohydrates

Sooner or later you will go off the Atkins diet. However, not planning ahead can mean weight regain, or worst of all, weight rebound, when you gain it all back and actually put on even more weight. It is possible due to the strong nature of sugar cravings and how even small amounts of simple carbs can re-wire the brain.

If you decide to go off low carb, remember that table sugar and honey are not the only culprits in terms of sugar addiction. It is important to understand the difference between simple and complex carbohydrates.

Most of us know cake, cookies and candy are bad for us. But many of us take bread, pizza, potatoes, pasta and rice - brown or white - for granted, as part of an American diet. The truth is they are also all high in carbs. In fact, some classify pizza as highly 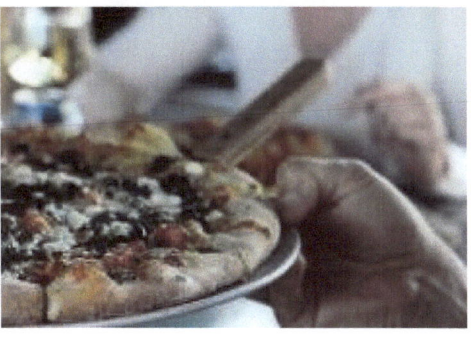 addictive because of all the carbs in the crust and in the tomato sauce, especially if they add sugar to it.

While it is true that brown rice and whole wheat products, for example, are complex carbohydrates, also referred to as 'slow carbs', as they are digested, they will break down into simple sugars before finally entering the blood stream.

Potato chips are considered to be as bad as, if not worse than candy, due to all of the (cheap) fat as well as carbs.

Foods that are high in carbs will be stored as fat if the energy from them, that is, the calories, are not burned. This leads to high triglyceride level and 'waist roundness', commonly referred to as a spare tire or a beer belly, in which most of the obese person's extra weight gathers around the middle. Triglycerides and waist roundness are 2 out of the 5 symptoms of metabolic syndrome, which is a forerunner of diabetes.

Controlling your insulin levels is one of the most important things you can do to optimize your overall health, and avoiding sugar and carbs is essential to doing this.

If you are going to eat them, work them off in one of two ways. The first is to burn as many, or more calories than you consume. A deficit of 500 calories per day will result in the loss of a pound of weight per week. The second way, in conjunction with the first, is to boost your metabolism so that your body will burn calories more efficiently and not store them as fat. You do this by building muscle through strength training.

In the detox program we outlined above, we included 2 forms of exercise, walking and yoga. We included this because they can be done by people any age, regardless of their fitness level in most cases. If you can stand on your own 2 feet, you can do both forms of workout.

Walking is an aerobic and cardio workout if you walk fast enough to be a bit breathless if you try to talk. The current recommendation is to walk 10,000 steps a day, about 3.5 to 5 miles, in order to meet the suggested daily level of activity.

Yoga twice a week will meet the suggested weekly activity of 2 strength-training sessions for about 30 minutes each. Yoga will help you build long, lean muscles, which will boost your metabolism.

An obvious benefit to both is that if you're busy doing them, you're much less likely to be eating. They will also boost energy, elevate mood, reduce stress, and help you get a good night's sleep.

You don't have to feel powerless in the face of sugar addiction. You can use this sugar detox program any time you think your bad habits are getting the better of you. Keep your journal to remind you of your success, so you can be your best self.

Final Thoughts

Now that an increasing body of research is pointing more and more to the addictive nature of sugar and high carbohydrate foods, if you feel that food cravings are running your life, it's time to take action to crack the sugar habit. Low carb and clean eating are the perfect way to detox and get your life and weight back under control.

Are You Ready For A Sugar Detox?

We have been talking throughout this book about how bad sugar is for your health and that you should to go through a sugar detox to break your sugar habit. And we provided a 15-day plan on how to do that.

But are you ready for it? I'll be honest with you, if you're consuming quite a bit of sugar each day (and who isn't?), this isn't going to be easy. Keep reading to make sure you know what you're in for, so you'll be prepared. That alone will help you tough it out and make it through your sugar detox days.

It Takes Willpower

It's going to take some willpower to make it through a sugar detox. You're going to want that candy bar or donut. Are you ready to not give in and make it through a few days of sugar cravings? The key is to keep in mind that it will get easier as time goes by and that you're doing this for an important reason - to improve your health, lose weight, look better, feel better and reduce your risk of developing Type II diabetes. Keep reminding yourself that you can do this and that it will be worth it in the end.

If you want it bad enough, you will find the willpower to make it through your sugar detox. Of course, keeping all sugar treats out of the house will help with temptation as well.

It's Not Going To Be Pleasant

This isn't going to be easy and it isn't going to be pleasant. In addition to craving your favorite sugary treats, you'll likely experience headaches and possibly nausea, joint pain and dizziness. Knowing this ahead of time will keep you from being shocked and surprised when these detox side effects start to pop up.

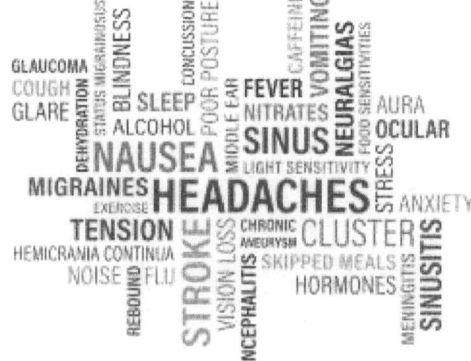

It helps to start your sugar detox on a Friday. You can make it through your work day before the headaches start and then have all weekend to detox. By the time Monday rolls around you should be through the worst of it. Just keep yourself busy or spend a good amount of time sleeping as you make it through to the other side.

The Side Effects Will Be Temporary And You'll Come Out Of It Feeling Much Better

Speaking of that, keep reminding yourself that this is only temporary. Make yourself tough it out one more hour, then one more, and one more ....

Go watch a movie, call a friend or go for a walk. Distract yourself and before you know it that hour will be over.

Keep it up hour after hour and you'll get through your sugar detox before you know it. Remember that this is only a temporary feeling. I promise that you'll feel much better after a few hours. The health benefits of freeing yourself from your sugar addiction are well worth the making it through the unpleasant side effects of a sugar detox. Because the addiction to sugar is much the same as it is to cocaine, the withdrawal symptoms will also be similar. Power through it and come out the other end a new person!

To your best self!

Other Relevant Books by This Author

If you would like to read more relevant books about this topic, here is a list of the CreateSpace links, titles and descriptions from this author:

https://www.createspace.com/6591616

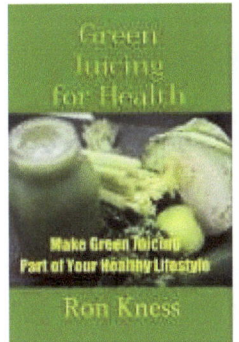

Green Juicing for Health

Green juicing, also known as vegetable juicing, combines a variety of leafy greens and other vegetables which are then processed through a juicer, instead of a blender.

In the fast-paced world today, time is the most precious commodity for most people, especially working professionals. In order to save time, they turn to processed foods, which include frozen meals and canned foods. They are convenient and easy to prepare.

However, eating too much processed foods could prove to be harmful for our bodies. They contain substantial amounts of saturated and trans-fats, i.e. unhealthy fats, along with sugar and salt. Prolonged intake of such foods causes people to fall sick easily. Coupled with stress in this society, it's no wonder diseases are more common and rampant among us today!

Health is wealth. As more people are becoming conscious of their health and total wellness, many have incorporated green juicing as part of their diets. It is easy to prepare and saves time. And what's more, the health benefits of green juicing are tremendous.

In my book, I cover how to add green juice to your diet as part of a healthy lifestyle, including a few recipes that taste great!

https://www.createspace.com/6471072

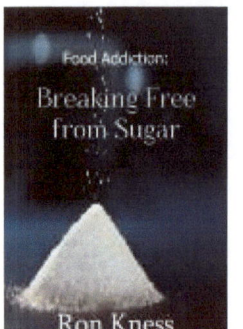

Food Addiction: Breaking Free from Sugar

The thought of eliminating sugar from your diet may seem like torture but actually, it is one of the healthiest things you can do for yourself. Processed sugar acts like a drug to the body adding no nutritional value to your diet - just empty calories.

Most people eat an enormous amount of sugar each day, usually in processed foods such as cereal and soft drinks. Processed sugar is thought to be contributing factor in health issues such as obesity, heart disease, and diabetes.

Each teaspoon of sugar contains 4 grams of sugar, which by the way equates to 16 calories. Most people eat more than 22 grams (5.5 teaspoons) of sugar each day.

Too much sugar can cause obesity, heart disease, liver damage, tooth decay and a whole host of other health conditions.

In this book we show you how to recognize hidden sugar, how to break free and detox from the addiction and reduce or eliminate sugar from your diet. Take control and break free from sugar!

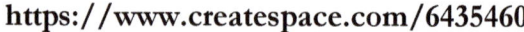

https://www.createspace.com/6435460

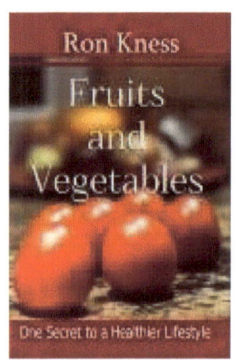

Fruits and Vegetables

The way the human body processes food has not changed for thousands of years, however, our predominant food supply has. With the advent of modern agricultural and food processing methods, we have seen a lock-and-step increase in heart disease, cancer and other dangerous and deadly conditions.

That is because modern-day food is unfortunately highly processed. Salt and refined sugar, monosodium glutamate (MSG) and trans fats, preservatives, steroids and man-made chemicals are intentionally injected into most of the food you eat.

This is not done to make you healthier. It is simply done to make the food longer on store shelves, taste better, and to produce as addictive a product as possible (so that you will buy more of it).

Fresh vegetables and fruits (not fried or slathered in unhealthy dressing) have naturally healthy levels of the nutrients, minerals and vitamins your body needs. They do not contain the processed sugar, insanely high levels of salt, steroids, preservatives and other nutritionally bankrupt chemicals found in processed food.

Unfortunately, the fruits and vegetables that human beings once used to eat in abundance are now lacking in most diets. Your body still craves the same nutrition requirements it did when your ancestors were eating healthy foods.

However, if you continue to reward your hunger with too much unhealthy processed food, and not enough healthy fruits and vegetables, poor health and debilitating medical conditions will be your reward.

The fact that you are a product of nature, and fruits and vegetables are natural food sources, reveals why they are so important as a part of your healthy diet plan.

Another important aspect of swapping out processed foods for vegetables and fruits has to do with how much you weigh. If you find it hard to lose weight and maintain a slim, trim, sexy figure, your diet is probably to blame.

In this book, we explore the fruits and vegetables you should be eating, how much of each you should be eating each day and share some tips on how to increase your fruit and vegetable consumption. Change your diet today and enjoy good health tomorrow and beyond!

https://www.createspace.com/6440684

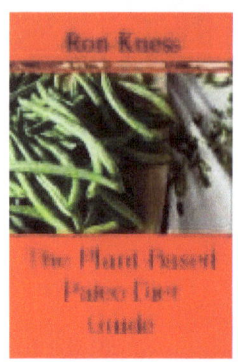

The Plant-Based Paleo Diet Guide

Have you heard about the caveman diet? Also known as the Paleo diet, it mimics the foods that humans ate during the Paleolithic era.

During this prehistoric era, humans ate whatever plants, fruits, vegetables and meats were available to them. That simple nutrition plan means that only natural foods entered their bodies.

Why is that important? Because scientists have studied the remains of humans from the Paleolithic time period, and found they didn't suffer from many of the diseases of today: diabetes, high blood pressure, cholesterol problems, obesity and heart disease.

In short our diet of today is killing us. But you can eat like they did and improve your health. I show you how in this book.

We start out by defining which foods are on and are not on this plant-based diet as a basis to start from. From there we go into some changes that people prescribing to veganism and some vegetarians will have to make to strictly adhere to their choice of eating.

We wrap up with a discussion of meat - the good and bad points, and if you should include it in your Paleo diet or not. After all our ancestors ate quite of bit of meat, but it wasn't commercially farm-raised.

Anyway, I think you will find this book informative and could be just what you are looking for if you are searching for a change from what you are eating now. Enjoy!

About the Author

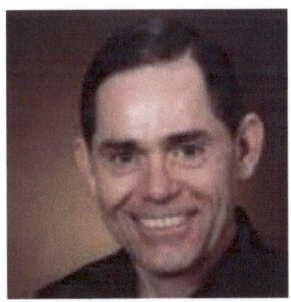

I grew up in Central Minnesota, where my parents owned and operated a fishing resort. Once out of high school I tried a couple of semesters of college, only to quit halfway through the Spring term; I decided at that time that college wasn't for me.

Then I decided to follow my father's previous occupation as an auto mechanic. I graduated from a two-year of vocational training course and worked as a mechanic for five years. While in vocational training, I decided to join the National Guard where I eventually ended up working full-time for 32 years.

So how does all of this relate to writing? In one of my leadership schools, the instructor, who was an English teacher at a juvenile detention center, presented writing to me in a whole new way - a way that started to develop my interest in working with words.

I eventually went back to college on the GI Bill while I was working and earned my Bachelor's degree in Business Administration. Taking a class or two per semester at night and on weekends took me seven years to complete my degree.

Fast forward about 40 years and I now have published over 100 books on Amazon for Kindle, CreateSpace and other publishing platforms.

Besides my own writing, I also ghostwrite ebooks, books, reports, articles, blogs and do Kindle conversions for clients on a variety of topics.

Today my wife and I are retired from our careers and live in Gold Canyon, AZ. I now write as a retirement business where you'll find me happily sitting in my office typing away on my laptop as I work on my next book or ghostwriting project . . . that is if we are not traveling on a cruise ship - our new-found mode of travel.

www.ingramcontent.com/pod-product-compliance
Lightning Source LLC
Chambersburg PA
CBHW050829290526
45792CB00001B/321